DON'T BURY ME...IT AIN'T OVER YET

CHARLES SCHNEIDER

Bloomington, IN Milton Keynes, UK

AuthorHouse™
1663 Liberty Drive, Suite 200
Bloomington, IN 47403
www.authorhouse.com
Phone: 1-800-839-8640

AuthorHouse™ UK Ltd.
500 Avebury Boulevard
Central Milton Keynes, MK9 2BE
www.authorhouse.co.uk
Phone: 08001974150

First published by AuthorHouse 2/23/2006

ISBN: 1-4259-1395-4 (sc)

Printed in the United States of America
Bloomington, Indiana

This book is printed on acid-free paper.

DEDICATION

This book is dedicated to my wonderful wife, who has continually stood by me for better or worse, and to the joys of my life: my son Charles IV and my daughter Melissa who have traveled with me through much of my restless soul's journey, and are responsible for providing me with my buddies: Christopher, Jessicca,, Samantha, Natalia, and Tyler. Lastly, I dedicate this book to all the victims of Alzheimer's disease and their caregivers. God bless every one of you.

INTRODUCTION

Here's the wind up... and the pitch... it looks like a curve ball... and he...

Life occasionally throws curve balls and I had just received a whopper. After working for thirty-five years, I was just five years away from retirement. Excited about all the great things I was going to do once I retired, but suddenly stopped cold by the news that I had a terminal disease. . I managed to pick myself up after the blow in a state of loss and confusion as to what I had just heard.

Only the good Lord knows our futures. I was only 52 years old when diagnosed with Alzheimer's disease; the thought of having Alzheimer's disease had never entered my mind before that moment. I was at the doctor's office to determine if I had Multiple Sclerosis when the doctor informed my wife and I that I had Alzheimer's disease.

Where did this come from?

I had lived the majority of my life teetering on the edge. I had tried to live everyday aware that it could be my last. And when Dr. Batchu informed me that I had,Probable, A.D., I figured the real "last day" was mighty close. Oddly enough, living the life of an "adrenalin junkie" for decades seemed to have help prepared me to deal with my new companion and would be possessor, Alzheimer's.

Now, because of my Alzheimer's, I am rarely tempted to seek out thrills to fulfill my need for excitement. My newly acquired disorder usually provides all the challenges that I need. For example, I can't think of any amusement park ride or thrill seeking activity that can reach down from the heavens, pick a person up, and redeposit him miles away from where he was just two seconds ago? Well, sometimes I find that I have been transported to strange places that I have no memory of. At times I have been contently sitting in a familiar spot when I was suddenly transported two hours ahead, or even behind, in time. Discovering that I suddenly occupy a foreign world is quite challenging.

Even if you do not presently know of anyone with Alzheimer's disease, I urge you to read this book and others about A.D. You will be amazed and appalled by this disease's capacity for destruction. Especially in Early Onset Alzheimer's, which usually strikes it's victims in their 20s to early 60s. If one lives beyond 85 years old their chances of getting this disease are near 50%. So it is likely that one day you may appreciate the knowledge you will gain by learning about A.D.

In this book you will read of good times, and heartbreaking times. I have endeavored to reduce the gloominess that I have found in much other literature about Alzheimer's disease, without trivializing the extent it mercilessly plagues its victims.

Personally, at this point of my life, I have not yet suffered the depression that so often accompanies Early Onset Alzheimer's Disease. I admit it provides many daily challenges, but then so does life in general. Being diagnosed with Alzheimer's disease is not cause to immediately start digging your grave. I intend on contributing more to this old world as long as possible. So please don't bury me! IT AIN'T OVER YET

CHAPTER 1
SO MUCH TO DO-
SO LITTLE TIME

I stood with my eyes locked on Dad's, seemingly lifeless body and saw this mountain of a man reduced to total helplessness. Mom turned toward me with tear filled eyes. Her body shook and her voice quivered as she said, "You're the man of the family now. Should we remove Dad's life support?

The doctor had informed us that there was little to no chance of Dad regaining consciousness. His heart had been severely damaged, his kidneys had stopped functioning, and he had undoubtedly incurred severe brain damage. I knew the right thing to do, but how could I order the final deathblow to the dad I loved so much? How could I take him away from all that he loved and all that loved him? Overwhelming grief and responsibility slammed down on me as I left the room knowing Dad was gone. I was 36 years old, not well myself, and not nearly as capable as Dad had been. I felt the overwhelming load that I had just inherited

1

from my father who had carried it for so long, and I felt so inadequate of assuming it.

Eighteen years have passed since Dad's departure. One year has passed since my diagnoses of Early Onset Alzheimer's disease.

My wife, Barb, and I are blessed with a daughter, Melissa 29, a son Charles 31, and 5 wonderful grandchildren ages 7 thru 13. I was approaching my retirement years and intended to spend a lot more time with our family. I had some health problems but nothing that would necessarily be fatal. I was having memory problems and was experiencing a lot of exhaustion. But the thought of having Alzheimer's Disease had never occurred to me. I had never even heard of Early Onset Alzheimer's Disease, so I didn't think Alzheimer's Disease could strike at my age. When the Doctor said based on my test results I have Early Onset Alzheimer's Disease.(E.O.A.D.) It took Barb and I totally by surprise. Soon after I was diagnosed, I started reading all I could find on E.O.A.D. I wanted to know exactly what I was up against.

I learned that E.O.A.D. usually strikes its victims in their 20's to early 60's and that it is considered the most aggressive form of A.D. The normal life expectancy is eight years after a diagnosis is made of A.D., but E.O.A.D. is usually considered to be more aggressive. There is a three stage and a seven stage scale used to describe the progression of A.D. I am using the three stage scale. The first stage generally lasts about 2 years, in which the victim can usually remain basically independent. During the second stage—which last from two to four years—the victim's independence erodes along with their capabilities. Knowing this, suggested to me that I had about two years of living relatively independently left. Allowing for E.O.A.D.'s aggressive nature and that I was diagnosed a year ago, it is possible for me to enter stage 2 at any moment. I felt pressured to get my personal and financial matters in order while I was still capable of doing so.

I took early disability retirement and applied for social security disability a few months ago.

I had made numerous promises before my diagnosis, and I wanted to keep them. I had promised my grandson, Chris, that I would take him fishing in the summer and let him operate the boat. I had promised Pat and Troy Perkins, Indian friends of mine, that I would bring another load of needed items to them on the Pine Ridge Reservation. I was determined to do everything I could to help my son get off to a good start on his marriage. I wanted to purchase a home where my wife could spend the rest of her life comfortably—with low maintenance and in a quiet neighborhood. There were a couple of projects I needed to complete for my mom. But the hardest thing I had yet to do was to prepare my family for what would soon occur.

There were legal and financial preparations to be made, but easing the emotional impact on my family was my toughest challenge. I wanted to spare my family the pain I felt when my dad died. I wasn't sure it was possible but I was going to try. I had spent much of my life trying to teach my children how to live and I felt that included showing them how to die when the time came. The more I learned about this horrid disease and how much it affects the family as well as the victim, the more I was determined to find a way to ease their pain. But how could I?

Barb is a strong woman, but I don't want to burden her with caring for a mindless body for a husband.

Just the thought of my body being used to insult or abuse my wife haunts me. I have been verbally abusive to her in past years and I have tried hard to make that up to her once I realized my mistakes. I can't bare the thought of ever subjecting her to that or any other type of abuse. I would truly rather die than to let that happen.

Yet, even my death would not solve the dilemma entirely. Barb would still have to deal with losing her husband prematurely. But each day I continue on living, I risk becoming possessed by the beast of E.O.A.D.. Holding me as his hostage, he could harass and abuse my beloved family. On days they didn't visit me, this ogre could inflict them with guilt, but on days they did

4

visit he could use my mouth to berate them. This intruder could choose to prolong my death, burdening my family, refusing them closure, locking them into caring for my mindless body. I would much prefer the destruction of this body over it being possessed and controlled by the likes of this beast.

I have faith in my Lord and Savior and am anxious to meet him.

Yet, I feel guilty when I think of leaving my loved ones so soon. I am willing to remain here as long as I possess the ability to be kind to my family. But if the time comes that I am no longer able to control my own actions, I pray the Lord will call me home.

CHAPTER 2
Life Altering Events

Many times, since my diagnosis, I find myself contemplating how I arrived to where I am today. I wonder if we are born with a certain amount of energy and have the ability to recharge as we wind our ways through life, similar to the way an automobile battery is recharged by an alternator. Certain conditions could cause the battery to weaken and die sooner, like overuse, extreme temperatures, or abuse--such as starting the car on a cold evening and immediately turning on the heater and the headlights. The alternator would work hard to fully recharge the battery while the automobile was draining it. Through aging and use, the battery eventually would weaken, or get enough dead cells that it no longer recharged as quickly or fully as it once did.

Navigating the trail of life requires constant energy.

Stressful situations require extreme amounts of energy. I think that some experiences are so severe that they not only temporarily drain us but also stifle future recharging sessions. I suspect that the accumulative effects of the Super Energy Drawing Events (S.E.D.E's) in my life have permanently minimized my ability to recharge. SEDE's may be, in part, or fully, responsible for the extreme fatigue that I have endured for years. Or perhaps it is in part, or all, due to Early Onset Alzheimer's Disease ?

Usually, empathy for a loved one's predicament drained me more than when I was the direct victim of some misfortune. I will point out some of the major SEDE's in my life, as I suspect these experiences have undoubtedly influenced my attitude toward life and how I deal with Early Onset Alzheimer's Disease.

CHAPTER 3
Learning to Live in a Man's World

My dad bought homes and remodeled them. Then he either sold them or rented them out. Dad was far too busy operating the business end of the company to physically work on the properties. I started working for my dad in the summers of my Jr. High School years. At times I worked with his brothers, who I preferred working with to the ex-convicts, alcoholics, and other degenerates my father used to obtain for cheap labor. My dad was consistent in that he not only preferred cheap labor but cheap properties as well, which were usually in high crime areas. The physical work was enjoyable to me, and I got along well with the other employees. Working in high crime areas didn't bother me, and I prided myself at 14 years old, being stronger than most of the adult men I worked with. I felt like I was becoming a man, and it felt great.

School became intolerable. I had the mental capability to succeed--the academics--but I could not cope with the social atmosphere. The behavior of many of the other students seemed immature and the teachers often responded by treating all of us as juveniles. I was also struggling with my own lack of self-confidence, and it contributed to my frustration with the school Environment. I had also recently abandoned my Christian beliefs creating a major void spiritually within myself.

To replace my crumbled belief system I created my own code of ethics. I needed an anchor to survive in the unstable world.

Mom and Dad assumed I was too lazy and stubborn to apply myself to schoolwork. I tried to make them understand the depth of my problems with school emotionally, but was unsuccessful. By the time I was fifteen I could no longer force myself to attend school for my parents' sake. I had long tried to gain their understanding to no avail, and I decided it was time to make a decision. I could not remain in their home defying their wishes daily by refusing to attend school. My self-made code of ethics, that I had attempted to replace my Christian values with, would still not allow me to disrespect my parents like that. It seemed that my only option was to leave home and start supporting myself. If I was going to make my own decisions, I should be mature enough to live on my own.

My best friend Doug had a cause for wanting to live on his own also. We wanted to go to Florida, but were forced to try Kentucky, our second choice, when we discovered that we didn't have enough money to afford tickets to Florida. Together we boarded the Greyhound bus toward a world full of possibilities. Things were looking pretty good after two days into our new lives. We had found jobs, and I figured I could afford a car in a couple of weeks. Our new lives lasted only three days. Dad discovered our whereabouts and immediately raced to Kentucky to get us. When Mom and Dad arrived, I tried to explain my dilemma and why I chose to leave. Although Dad did not really understand my logic, he agreed to let me quit school and start working fulltime.

I returned home and obtained a full time job in a warehouse. I scored very high on their pre-employment test, and they asked me to work in the office. But I feared the office job would be too similar to a school environment, so I opted for a laborer position in the warehouse instead.

I was visiting a friend in my old neighborhood when I decided to stop by our previous home and chat with the new owners who were friends of our family. When I knocked on the door of 124 South Clark Ave. I had no clue that my life was about to change forever. My intentions were only to chat with the family briefly. Instead, I left there with a life long companion. This bubbly, compassionate sixteen-year-old would lead me to joy I never thought possible. Thirty-six years later I sometimes have to hold back tears when I think of the love and commitment she has given me. She took me--a young man who had never felt loved--and gave me her unconditional love. August 3, 1968 we were married. Today I'm so thankful that we had the courage to do what we knew was right even though no one else agreed with us at the time. I don't recommend getting married that young, but we were both mature beyond our years and for us it was definitely the right thing to do.

We started out with a beat up 1960 Chevy car, a couple of hundred dollars, and a minimal amount of furnishings. At 16 years old I could not legally sign a marriage license without parental consent or sign a lease agreement. My dad knew me well enough to know that if my mind was set, I was going to get married and we would need a place to live. So he went along and signed for me to get married and signed the apartment lease agreement for us. It took very little to satisfy Barb and I. We were so in love that not much else mattered to us. Soon after we were married I entered a partnership with my neighbor Paul painting houses. After a few months of painting houses I received and accepted a proposition from Dad. We agreed that I would remodel homes that he bought, and he would pay me $75.00 a week, as a draw, against 50% of the profit when he sold the houses. It was easy to convince me. I had always dreamed of a father and son business. Now, it would be a reality!

We started with an old 2-story house that was severely fire damaged. The roof was burnt thru, windows all broken out, and much of the siding was gone. Almost all of the interior walls and ceilings were burnt or smoke covered. There was water damage from the Fire Dept. suppressing the flames and from the recent rains.

Living on $75 a week was a struggle, but we decided that we could squeeze by until we received our share of the profits. We both wanted a puppy but when we added one to our family the apartment manager didn't approve. We had to get rid of Trix or move. We decided to move into the burnt home, where we could keep our puppy and save on rent temporarily. The house needed extensive framing work and I had little experience at that level, but I was a fast learner. So dad would come by once or twice a day and advise me how to do things. Along side me was my ever willing wife and our faithful companion, Trix. Trix was a very intelligent dog and he quickly learned to climb the ladder so that he could be with us while we worked on the roof. We were an inseperable three- some

Winter came and the cold wind blew snow into the house through the cracks in the walls and the boarded up windows. I truly regret how insensitive I was to Barb's needs. Like heat! It did not seem that bad to me. But for Barb, 20 to 30 degrees with snow blowing into the house was unbearable. After coming to my senses, I took Barb over to my parent's house to thaw her out, but that was just a temporary solution, so we made some adjustments to the old house to make it bearable. Barb's little sister, Patty, was going to stay with us for a while. So we put our mattress on the large bathroom floor, where we could stay warm while we slept. We made a bed for Patty in the tub. Barb used the only working electrical outlet to cook our meals with a hotplate. We had to shuttle in 5 gallon buckets of water from my parent's house. Despite our difficult circumstances we were happy and still so much in love. I often lost my temper when things didn't go as planned with the repairs, and Barb just patiently continued to help as best she could. What a fool I was to ventilate my anger towards Barb that way. I have tried so hard to make amends to her. She did her best to tolerate my independent and angry ways. She would tell me I'm just her untamed Wildman. I don't have much anger anymore but I retained my independent, and many times, unorthodox ways.

Since we lived there, we worked seven days a week, only taking off to eat and sleep. Life wasn't easy. But it was good, and we were surviving on our $75 weekly allowance. After 7 or 8 months we were nearly completed with the house's remodeling. We had to find another place to live so Dad could sell this one and give Barb and I our share of the profits.

Dad owned a small house that he agreed to arrange financing on if we purchased it from him. So for the price of $8,900 we purchased our first home. I remodeled another house in partnership with Dad and continued taking a $75 per week draw. Now that we had house payments it was extremely hard to survive on my weekly draw. The first house sold while I was remodeling the second house, but Dad did not speak with me about splitting the profits. I figured he was too busy and might still be working out the numbers. I didn't ask him about it.

I completed the second house a couple of months later, and it sold quickly. I waited a week or two for Dad to pay me my share of the profits on both houses, but he still did not offer it. When I finally approached him about it, he simply said that there was no profit in either of them. I did not believe him. I had some idea of what he paid for them and how much my pay and the material costs were. By my calculations, there were many thousands of dollars left as profit, but I loved and respected my dad too much to pursue the matter any further. My mind now digresses to past times of Dad doing smaller but similar things to me before and after that time.

I had already realized that the world was not a perfect place, but I still wasn't prepared to deal with my own father cheating me out of money that he would not have even missed. It wasn't because of the financial loss, but rather the realization that the dad I loved so much could act as if he cared so little for me. Maybe I felt as sorry for him as I did for myself. I wanted to cry, but by then I was too hardened to allow tears. Even though Dad was a wonderful man and redeemed himself many times after that incident, I still think a part of me died that day. It was one of those super energy-drawing events. It left a part of me unable to ever recharge.

CHAPTER 4
Losing Our Child

We couldn't continue to live on $75.oo a week so I sought a better job. Being seventeen made it hard for me to get a job that paid enough for us to live on. But I was determined to find a way. I looked older than I was and could easily pass for 25 to 30, so I used that to my advantage.

There was a real estate management company in a depressed area in St. Louis. They managed over 5,000 rental units and had difficulty acquiring and retaining good help. They paid reasonably well, but I would have to risk being robbed or killed in the areas they required me to work in. I started at more than twice the pay I had been earning and was given plenty of overtime opportunities. I knew I had to look and act tough to survive the area I worked in. So I took the appropriate steps. I grew a mustache, bought me a cowboy hat, and took up smoking cigars. Combining that with my 5'11" 200 pound muscular body and the ability to lift the front end of a car, I felt I was prepared to survive.

My wife and I were living in our own home, driving a take home van from my employer, and making good money. We had Trix and each other, and it seemed that life was as good as it could ever be. Soon I was foreman over a group of ex-convicts, freshly released mental patients, and some common, but desperate, people. Part of my duties required me to go into many dangerous places alone, and there were some very scary situations. But I refused to let fear keep me from supporting my wife. Things just seemed to keep getting better and better for us.

After being married for three years, we felt it was time to add a child to our family. As foster parents, we were prepared to take advantage of an unusual situation. A woman we knew, Marlene, had several children inside the foster care system. Her youngest was a one-year-old and living with her, but she needed to find a good family that could adopt her baby. Marlene didn't feel she had the resources to raise Jessica adequately, and it hurt her to see what was happening to her older children as they were moved from one foster home to another. Marlene selected Barb and I to be Jessica's adoptive parents. We took physical custody of Jessica while the adoption was proceeding through the legal system. Barb and I instantly fell in love with our precious little "Ka-Ka," as she called herself. Her curly brown hair and bright smile just melted us. We showered her with love and gifts during the six months that she stayed with us.

The adoption procedure was almost finalized when our hearts were broken. The Department of Social Services informed us that they technically had legal custody of Jessica, and they demanded she be immediately removed from our home and placed in another temporary foster home. Since we were already one of the foster home options for the Department of Social Services we requested that they allow us to be her temporary foster parents until the adoption was complete. The caseworker said that it was against their policy to allow pending adoptee parents to have custody of the child during the adoption process. We told the caseworker that Jessica had already been bounced around from home to home and we thought it made sense for Jessica to remain in her current home until any decision was made. The caseworker insisted she would come over that night to pick up Jessica.

Having no choice in the matter, we packed Jessica's things and prepared for her to leave. When the case worker arrived we told her that we had purchased several birthday presents for Jessica's two year old birthday and asked if she would take them to Jessica's new temporary home to be opened on her birthday, next week. We could not believe our ears when the caseworker rudely refused to allow Jessica to keep the gifts. It seemed she was angry with us and we didn't understand why. Barb and I were so hurt for the heartless treatment they were subjecting our baby daughter to. I do still remember the heart-wrenching pain of having our daughter pulled from Barbs loving arms and carried away by a seemingly cold hearted, insensitive agent of the government.

I went down to the Social Services office thinking I could easily correct whatever resentment they had toward us. The caseworker's supervisor restated that policy required Jessica be removed from our home because we wanted to adopt her. I was angry and frustrated at how ridiculous it was to subject Jessica to more foster homes and how offensive it was to deny her a birthday gift. I pointed out that it seemed as if they were not interested in Jessica's needs. She angrily shouted back to me, "You tried to work outside of our system and we will not allow you to have Jessica." My heart was broken from losing Jessica and it was broken for little Ka-Ka losing permanent parents who truly loved her. But I think what broke my heart the most was seeing Barb's heart so completely broken. I felt so inadequate and guilty for letting Barb and Ka-Ka down.

It is just incomprehensible to me that human beings could deliberately sabotage a child's life for their own self-serving interests. These are people who are paid to help children and to build trust with them! Learning what many of them were really like revealed further how pitiful and self-serving people can often be. I would like to believe that this was just a freak, evil incident, but I have seen too many examples of this type of selfish behavior in others: law enforcement, medical field, attorneys, school teachers, ministers. It seems logical to assume that these occupations would be chosen by people whose primary wish was to serve others. Unfortunately for me, I've seen too much to believe in that myth.

Knowing that Social Services had legal custody of Jessica, and that they would never agree to let us have her back, or adopt her, we had to accept the cold hard fact that we had lost her from our lives. We still hold her in our hearts. Many times I have pulled her picture out to see her again and wonder how she is doing. Jessica would be in her early thirties now and if our many prayers for her have been answered, I'm sure she is doing well. This Super Energy Drawing Event took a chunk of our hearts and lives. Earlier I said that a part of us dies as a result of these type incidents, but I think more accurately is that a part of our will to live dies.

Within the next three years God blessed us with two children, and we raised them alongside numerous other children who were temporarily troubled or homeless. We took in children on our own, no longer through Social Services, and hopefully blessed their lives. They were a blessing to us. It may be an often dark, self-serving world, but by refusing to conform, and doing the right thing, we have been so blessed with inner peace.

CHAPTER 5
Attack of the unknown

It was my sixth year as a police officer. I was fired up and committed to stopping crime. I loved my job as patrolman and detective. I was admired and respected by most of the other officers. I brought in felony arrests almost daily. I worked hard at building my reputation as being fair but firm. I was practically fearless and extremely confident. But internal pressure was increasing, and soon it would change my life.

The County we lived in was starting forced bussing. That meant my children, 7 and 9 years old, could be bussed to an inner city school. A dangerous high crime area! I had been exposed to enough high crime areas, working two jobs so that I could raise my children in the suburbs. Now the government was telling me I had to surrender my authority over that part of my children's lives, let them be forcibly bussed into a high crime area. We had already lost one child due to government intrusion and I was not going to let it happen again. Only over my dead body. I wondered how this could be happening in our free country? I discussed this matter with Barb and told her of my strong feelings. Barb agreed that we should not let this happen. We considered staying in the school district and simply refuse to comply, but we ultimately chose another option, to move to another County.

There was a nice town about 200 miles away hiring Police Officers from the St. Louis area to obtain their experience. We decided to move there, confident that I would be able to join the police department once we had settled there. But right after we relocated, they activated a hiring freeze due to budget cuts. It was a bad situation, but we would just have to wait it out. I stayed in my parent's home during work days and returned to my family on my off days, or they drove in to visit me. We lived that way for one year, expecting the hiring freeze to be de-activated. This type of situation was a nightmare for a man whose life revolved around his family, and was taking an extremely large toll on me.

A second highly stressful situation came also. My dad went to my sister's aid to change a flat tire. He parked his car behind my sister, Kim's, car on a curvy section of a snow-covered road. My Dad saw a police car parked about a block away and hoped the police officer would realize the danger of the situation and assist them. Instead he just remained where he was parked and watched as a truck slid around the curve, crashing into dad's car and crushing dad's legs between his car and Kim's car. With Dad's diabetes and heart condition, the effects of the broken leg were compounded. He suffered through a year filled with operations. I was already stressed from having to spend most of my time 200 miles away from Barb and our children. Now, I was very worried about dad too. Then another extremely stressful situation hit me.

The acting Police Chief of the department I was employed by was a well-liked personable fellow. I considered him a friend. Then the bomb hit! An informant told me the acting Police Chief, who will remain nameless, had molested a young mentally handicapped girl. He told me that he knew none of us would do anything about it because police always stick together. He was wrong. There was no way I would ignore something like this, if it was true. I needed to know and looked into the allegations. After speaking to the little girl and her parents, I suspected the allegations were true. There were some complicating factors occurring within the police department and city council at the time. Some of the councilman wanted the acting chief to become the permanent police chief even after knowing what he had done. As politics entered, and considering the fact that it's not easy to investigate your own superior officer, I decided to solicit outside help. Boy was I in for another shock!

I contacted the F.B.I. and explained the situation to them. The F.B.I. agent told me he was not interested, the F.B.I. did not investigate things like that. I responded, you investigate civil rights violations, such as a police officer assaulting someone, and this is a case of an on duty police officer sexually assaulting a young retarded child. The unconcerned Federal Agent just repeated his refusal to become involved. I then contacted the county sex crimes division. After explaining the entire situation to them, they said that unless the victim initiated a complaint they would not become involved. I reminded them that part of their job was to investigate. But still, they refused to help. I was angry and devastated. I stubbornly dove into the investigation at my own risk. This was an extremely stressful situation for me. Along with being away from my family and worried about Dad, it was more than I could take. This was a real super energy drawing event. The stress increased when I found out that there were many more young children this predator had molested. Eventually he was convicted of seven felony charges, resulting in some Alderman seeking revenge against me.

One year later the hiring freeze was still in effect. We decided not to wait any

longer and relocated to a fast-growing county without "bussing," neighboring the county of my place of employment. Dad was doing better, but still in pretty bad condition. I got a letter a few months later, advising me the hiring freeze had been de-activated. Too late for that now!

Getting settled in our new home, I went outside to do some yard work. Suddenly I collapsed to the ground exhausted. After lying there a while, I gathered up the strength to get up. I went into the house and sat down at the dining room table. I had been very tired before, but had never felt so weak and exhausted as I did then.

On my off days from the police department I owned and operated a remodeling company. Having committed to bid some work at a friends house, I forced myself up and headed for his house. My weakness persisted and I became dizzy and faint. Shortly after I arrived at my friend's house, he drove me to the hospital. After scaring the heck out of Barb, and several hours of tests and hospital rest, I was told they could find nothing wrong with me. I was feeling much better, so Barb drove us home. What had happened to me? A couple of days later, while I was on duty, the dizziness and weakness returned. This time it brought a panic type fear with it. I considered myself a rock, almost totally fearless. What in the world was happening to me? The condition continued to come and go every other day or so. One doctor diagnosed me as "lactose intolerant," while another doctor diagnosed it as "panic attacks." I had no idea what was happening to me. For about a year I struggled with this condition. I lost strength, my vision declined, I was extremely fatigued , I had major short and long-term memory loss and my mind felt like it was in a great fog. I forced myself to work my police job, but had to give up my remodeling work. I could no longer enthusiastically perform my police duties. I had to force myself just to do the minimum necessary tasks. I still don't know what was wrong with me. But I knew my family needed me, so I kept pushing on. I started wondering if I had a fatal disease, or if I was losing my mind. I repeatedly begged God to let me last long enough to raise my children. After about a year of living with this condition, too weak to fight on, I finally turned it all over to God. I told God that I thought my family needed me, but you are wiser than I am, so if it's your will that I die or go crazy, I'll accept it. I started getting better shortly after that and have remained ever grateful, for being given the wonderful blessing of being allowed to go on raising our children.

I believe that making memories is far more important than accumulating an excess amount of material things that never last forever. I intended, the precious times we had spent memory making, to last forever in all of our minds. All those family vacations, sitting together in front of the fireplace with the kids, their first steps, and so many others, are mostly gone now. Some unidentified evil has stolen them from me. If it had been a common thief, I would have hunted him down, no matter how long it took. I would never quit until I found a way to force him to give back my most prized possessions, my memories. I had to harness my anger, hurt, and frustrations and apply all I had left to providing, what I still could, for my family. They still deserved the love, protection and financial support of their father, and husband .But its not over, I will eventually overcome this beastly thief and retrieve my precious memories. I believe they are somehow recorded in my Soul. When I step into eternity I'll have them all again. What a day that will be! In the meantime I'll go on making memories in every way still possible as long as possible.

Chapter 6
Welcome Home Son

If it is possible to love your children too much, I did. I still do. My wife and children were my life. I was determined to be the best father ever. If I was a great father, maybe I could spare my children the painful childhood and adolescence I had experienced. Despite my best efforts, I failed. When they withdrew their trust in me, I was devastated. Barb and I had differing opinions on how to handle our teenagers. We experienced stress in our marriage to the point that I almost lost her. This was definitely one of those S.E.D.E. times.

Knowing how easily my life could crumble, and that I could so easily lose the ones I loved so much, destroyed my sense of security and left a gaping wound in my heart.

The last S.E.D.E. I need to mention started with a telephone call from my son. He had been on his own several years. He didn't understand how much I loved him. I tried to use every opportunity I could to reach out to him. I continued to hope and pray that he would understand sometime. When he called, it was to ask if he could come stay with us a while and I readily invited him home. I was not prepared for what I saw when he entered our home. My handsome, strong, healthy son looked as beaten down as anyone I had ever seen. The pain and brokenness that radiated from him was indescribable, with his whole body shaking, his voice so weak, and his will defeated. I felt so sorry for him that I could barely keep standing. I don't think I'll ever get over the grief I felt for him that day. The realization that this often times terrible cruel world could inflict such pain and suffering on our son, Charley, took a chunk out of my heart that day. Of all the hurt and pain I have ever experienced, I believe this one hurt the most. To this day just the memory of it can bring tears to my eyes. I sometimes think about how God endured the great suffering of his son and feel like I can relate to how he must of felt then in my own small way.

CHAPTER 7
Why Me?

Other members of my AD group have asked, "Why me? Why do I have to be the one with Alzheimer's?" Out of 250 million people, why do I have to be one of the 4 million with A.D.? The odds of having A.D. are 62.5 to 1. Why am I so lucky? For those of us with Early Onset A.D. the odds are 1250 to 1. If you live to be 84 years old, your chances of getting A.D. are 1 in 4. Allow for the fact that the average life expectancy has been increasing and consequently many more will live past 84 years of age, and the odds of getting AD could rapidly increase to above 50%. I surely don't claim to know why some get Alzheimer's and others don't. Technically speaking, there are genetic causes and pre-disposition factors. I think eventually it will be proven that Alzheimer's is a group of diseases, and that there are many types of Alzheimer's and many different effects of each type.

Our understanding of Alzheimer's disease and other brain diseases are in their infancy stage. What we know of Alzheimer's today is about the equivalent of what Lewis and Clark knew about the land included in the Louisiana Purchase after one trip through it. There are still vast areas of the brain that have not been explored. If the Lord tarries the answers will probably be provided eventually. My heart breaks for many good people and their families that I know with this beastly disease, and hopefully help is soon coming.

Personally, I feel I am coping with my diagnosis and condition pretty well to this point. I am not sure that I know why. It could be because I have already been face to face with death so many times as I have witnessed many deaths and have been in many life threatening situations. Perhaps this has pre-conditioned me for a trauma like being diagnosed and living with Alzheimer's. Maybe it's just that my diagnosis came early and I have not deteriorated enough to experience the depression and fear that it so often brings, or maybe I am still in shock with the idea that this has happened to me. Or could it be because of the experience in my early 30's? I really don't know what happened to me then. Was it a nervous breakdown? Was it simply Panic Attacks? Or was it an exacerbation of M.S. Disease (which I have not been officially diagnosed with yet), or was it the beginning of Alzheimer's? Whatever it was, it struck me in the prime of my life and some of its effects have lasted till now. I felt like I was going to die, or worse, that I might become a terrible burden to my family by losing my mind. God is so gracious he spared me of enough of its effects that I was able to recover enough to be there and provide for my young family. In a way I feel like I've been on extended time since then. Maybe that helps me to accept and deal with the Alzheimer's now.

Here is another possible explanation for why I am not yet depressed or fearful about Alzheimer's. Could it be that I have so many physical ailments, like sleep apnea, or diabetes, or high blood pressure, that I am somewhat wore down and closer to accepting death. Or maybe it's because I simply have put my trust in God. Let me tell you, heaven does sound mighty fine! But I do know that I want to use whatever time and capabilities I have left to help others as much as I can. Hopefully in some small way I can encourage caregivers, AD victims, and all of those seeking a cure for Alzheimer's.

CHAPTER 8
Restless Soul

I have had a full life during which time I've had three primary occupations.   Carpentry, law enforcement, and firefighting along with emergency medical technician. Please bear with me on what I am about to say. I am not writing about my past to brag or complain. I included it because I have been helped so much by reading books by authors with Early Onset Alzheimer's Disease, largely because of their complete honesty and openness about themselves and their individual situation. I want to be as thorough and open as they were. I have been a restless soul most of my life. As a result Barb and I have lived in approximately thirty homes. I have a saying about my life, "I have failed at more things, than most people have ever tried." Before going any further I would like to clarify how it is possible for me to write so much about the past if I lost so much of my long-term memory.

I am using several forms of information gathering. I am tapping in to my wife's memory and referring to business records, copies of police reports, family pictures, old home movies, and other resources. I am also using my long-term memory. It's strange how Alzheimer's affects its victims. At certain times I can remember much more than at another time. This seems to be common among victims of Alzheimer's. It seems to me, if the brain is actually destroyed in areas, as autopsies reveal, that this occasional increase in recall should not be possible. Maybe I'll address this mystery later. However, I do actually recall much of what I have written about. My long-term memories are sort of fragmented and most specifics erased. An example of this is how I remember taking our children to Disney World. I thought we had only gone there once until Barb reminded me that we had been there twice. After she reminded me, I vaguely remembered a second trip, but I can't recall any of the details, like what we did or where we went, what rides we rode, which ones the kids liked, where we stayed, or how old our children were. The specific happenings, like when the kids displayed their joy, are all missing. This type of puzzle is why I am so thankful for others who wrote so honestly about their experiences with AD. Perhaps through comparing notes and understanding things like this cat-and-mouse type functioning of the brain it can help lead us to a cure. So here is a brief summary of my past.

Besides performing multiple duties and holding numerous positions in the capacity of my three primary careers, I have owned and operated several businesses, worked as, and voluntarily participated in, many things. The businesses include a fencing company, a roofing company, a building and remodeling company, and two private investigative companies. I worked as a warehouse material handler, a carpenter, a maintenance man, a construction foreman, a security guard, a salesman, a house painter and a certified hypnotherapist. I was a Sunday school teacher, an assistant youth director, a counselor, a short-term missionary, a Bible smuggler, and the host of a radio talk show. I have been fortunate enough to have traveled to numerous countries on five continents, and to most of the fifty states. I have lost my home and personal possessions to an airplane crash at the age of 5years old. Barb, the children, and I have lost our home and possessions to a flood, and another home to a bankruptcy. I have been asked many times, "how does Barb put up with you?" I have also been told many times that my wife must be a saint! I think she just understands me and loves me that much! There are still many places I have not been and many things I've never tried. But now, I no longer have much desire to do many of them. My full life has provided many experiences. I have been attacked with knives (the first time, at 5 years old), have been involved in hundreds of fist fights, hit by a car, shot at, made over 1,000 arrests, been severely burned, observed the deaths of fellow officers, watched a man trapped inside a burning car die before we could rescue him, saw gunshot victims die on the street , been knocked out by a 2x4, had people attempt to kill me numerous times, ran over by a truck and harassed by a KBG officer in Russia. I have been tied up and locked in a closet, watched an eleven-year-old die on the street, seen brothers attack brothers, stood helplessly as a lady died because I hadn't been properly trained on how to help her. Have been hunted by police in China, and attacked with chains and bricks. I have watched children see their mom die a horrid death on the city streets. I have had my life threatened more times than I could recall—even if I didn't have AD

As for my heath experiences, I have Arthritis, Diabetes, Hypothyroidism, Sleep Apnea, Spinal Stenosis, Essential Tremors, Restless Leg Syndrome, double vision that comes and goes, a broken foot that has only partially healed. I am overweight, bleed excessively from a tiny scratch and possibly have multiple sclerosis.

This partially describes who I am, who I was, but not really, because this only describes what I have endured and experienced not how I viewed it or handled it. However, my past has undoubtedly affected how I reacted to having AD. Please excuse me for not giving details of the many incidents and involvements due to the urgency I feel to complete this book.

CHAPTER 9
Alzheimer's, Who are You?

Before I was diagnosed with Early Onset Alzheimer's disease, I thought there was only one type of Alzheimer's disease. I was totally unaware of the Early Onset type of Alzheimer's, which can strike people in their thirties, and possibly even in their twenties or younger. Most often it strikes people in their forties, and fifties, and possibly early sixties. It is estimated that there are 200,000 of us with EOAD in the U.S. That's an average of 4,000 per state. The area served by the St. Louis Mo. chapter of the Alzheimer's Association consist of about two million people. That's equal to about fifty percent of Missouri's population. Missouri, having about the same population as the average of other states, should have approximately 2,000 Early Onset victims in the St. Louis chapter area. Where are all the Early Onset victims? I have only been able to locate a dozen or so in our area. That leaves about 1,988 Early Onset Alzheimer's victims that I have not been able to locate. Perhaps good portions, say half of them, are in nursing homes. That still leaves about 994 victims of Early Onset Alzheimer's living in the St. Louis, Mo. Alzheimer's Association's area, probably struggling alone with their caregivers, receiving little or no help from the Alzheimer's Association. I have benefited greatly from my involvement with the Alzheimer's Association and by talking and sharing with those who are also victims of Early Onset Alzheimer's. It has been very encouraging to share with others in the same situation as myself.

DASNI is an international organization that provides a CHAT room at 3pm and 9pm Eastern Time, seven days a week .It is another great source of communication amongst A.D. victims. I have met some great people form all around the world through their CHAT room. I think that other victims of Early Onset Alzheimer's Disease and A.D. would benefit from DASNI, but it is hard to find and inform them of this option.

Early Onset Alzheimer's Disease is believed to be hereditary. It is often linked to genetic defects on three chromosomes. The more common form of A.D., which generally strikes its victims in their mid to late 60's and above, has been linked to an inherited protein called APOE. The three types of APOE proteins are, APOE2, APOE3, and APOE4. People who inherit APOE4 are more likely to be victims of A.D. after age 65. However, I have been diagnosed with the Early Onset type so I suppose the APOE4 I inherited is irrelevant. I have not been tested for the genetic defects that cause Early Onset Alzheimer's. This testing is expensive and unnecessary for me since I have already been diagnosed with the disease. The testing for the genetic defects, that affect three chromosomes, is only helpful about 50% of the time. The other 50% of people with Early Onset Alzheimer's disease may have defects on other chromosomes that have not yet been identified.

It is believed that Early Onset Alzheimer's disease not only strikes it's victims at a younger age, but that it is also a more aggressive form of the disease. Often victims of Early Onset Alzheimer's are diagnosed in the first stage of the disease since they are usually still employed and they notice the disease affecting their job performances. They are often forced to leave their jobs while in their 40's and 50's, or younger, some while still raising children. Because the spouse is usually the caregiver, he/she will have less time to offer the children and may have to leave his job in order to care for the afflicted spouse. Early Onset Alzheimer's Disease victims may have the added guilt and frustration of not being able to provide for and help out their family as they previously could.

Stage one Alzheimer's disease usually lasts about 2 years. Generally a person in Stage one can safely be alone for extended periods of time. Stage 2, the victim can perform some tasks but may need help on others. They forget words and what they are saying in mid-sentence occasionally. Depression, irritability and restlessness usually occurs. They are clearly becoming disabled and are aware of their severe deterioration. This can frustrate and depress the victim deeper. Short-term memory further decreases and orientation to time and place becomes clouded. Familiar faces may not be recognized. I think I may have entered into the early part of stage 2 now. Stage 2 of Alzheimer's Disease generally last about 2 years. Stage 3 is the last and final stage. It last from two to four years usually. However it has been known to last as many as 10 to 15 years. By stage three of Alzheimer's disease, I do not consider it a blessing to live any longer than the usual two to four years. In fact even one day of living with stage three of Alzheimer's disease is too much. It is my prayer that the Lord calls me home before Stage 3 of Alzheimer' Disease has taken over my mind. If I lasted to this stage I might not recognize anyone or be able to talk. I would need constant care, and would start developing severe physical complications. The physical complications become so critical the victim eventually dies. It is almost like the victim has left but the body stayed behind. Often AD patients become paranoid, aggressive, and insulting. I can only pray that my family be spared of that terrible possibility.

AD changes its victim's personality. It does not ask permission. It can change your language, steal any words it wants to, and give you profanity in their place. It can cast a spell of fear and hopelessness on many of its victims. It is not content to slowly kill you. It wants to torture, humiliate, embarrass, and confine you. It refuses to ease your suffering by allowing a quick death. It not only delights at abusing its victim, it also wants to torture their loved ones. A particular evil is that the more the family loves the AD victim, the more the predator can hurt them.

I think A.D. personifies many of this world's evils. It can create illusions or cause something right in front of your eyes to disappear or transform into something else. It can instantly transport you from where you are to another place and leave you wondering where you are and why you're there. It can often fill you with terrible guilt or fill you with fear and confusion. It can attack you, unseen, as often as it so desires. I wonder if it delights in the fact that its victims have no ability to retaliate. It is invisible and intangible. It destroys families, breaks hearts, and can destroy you financially .In late stages it can make your love transform into hate of your loved ones, cause us to falsely accuse them, and even abuse them. It deliberately procrastinates killing you, so it has time to destroy your very essence. It takes away your cherished memories and eliminates your ability to create more. I sometimes wonder how one's spirit and soul are responding as this alien intruder possesses our body.

There are some things beneficial to be said of A.D. however. It is not usually physically painful. Being diagnosed with it helps us realize what truly is important. It can trigger a spiritual arousing within us, and it allows us some time to prepare for its coming onslaught. I am reminded of a statement Job made. He had lost his children and all his wealth. Then he was afflicted with an extremely painful and grotesque disease and he responded by saying "Though he slay me I will trust in him." I feel the same way now, but I suspect if my brain continues to deteriorate, I might lose my ability to feel that way. Another benefit I have received because of A.D. is a sense of freedom. I can do what I want to, with little fear of failure. Perhaps it is because I am near the bottom already and have less to lose.

CHAPTER 10
What Are My Options?

There are four FDA approved drugs for people with, first stage, mild Alzheimer's disease. These drugs are Aricept, Cognex, Excelone, and Reminyl. They all slow the metabolic breakdown of acetylcholine, which is the brain chemical that helps cells communicate. Namenda is the only drug available for the moderate (stage 2) phase of Alzheimer's disease. It appears to protect the nerve cells, in the brain, against excess glutamate. Glutamate is a messenger chemical released from cells. No one knows exactly what causes Alzheimer's disease. There is speculation that head injuries may trigger the process, or that toxic chemicals are in part responsible. Some researchers suspect that Alzheimer's disease is a normal consequence of aging, and if everyone lived to be 120 or longer they would all get Alzheimer's disease. According to that theory some of our brains age prematurely giving us the disease, at a much earlier age than 120 years old. All of the drugs available for Alzheimer's disease only help control symptoms of the disease, and do not cure the disease or stop its progression. Some believe that Vitamin E and Ginkgo Biloba help treat the symptoms of Alzheimer's disease.

The estimated cost of Alzheimer's disease in the U.S. is between 80 to 100 billion dollars a year and increasing rapidly as the baby boom generation ages. The federal government recently doubled the amount allocated for research, which will help. But there are still many research projects that cannot be funded. The government seems to be more concerned about Alzheimer's disease now that it has become apparent that when the baby boomers start getting Alzheimer's disease, it will eventually break the health care system. Many consider Alzheimer's disease the worst disease available. I don't know if it is, or not .But I do believe their opinion is based on many true observations that surely provide some justification to believe as they do. At this time there are really no satisfactory medical options available, but there are some encouraging drugs being tested and researchers are learning more about A.D. daily. While those of us with A.D. have no option but to wait for a cure, we do have a choice, at least in the early stages, to how we react personally to A.D.I am presently reacting to it by endeavoring to stay as active as possible, to resist its progress to the best of my ability, and remain as positive as I can.

CHAPTER 11
What is it like to have Alzheimer's?

I would like to convey how I feel toward this disease and how it has affected my life. I constantly have the feeling that I am in slow motion. I not only think slower but I move slower also. I am like the proverbial turtle: I get there, just slowly, like when you first learned to drive, and you had to deliberately concentrate on keeping the car between the lines on the road. There was a lot to remember at the time, to check your speed, to remember which pedal was for the gas and which one was for the brake—throw in a clutch and you really had to think about where your feet were; if you mixed them up you could end up with lots of problems. At the same time you had to be attentive to other vehicles, road signs, people on the sidewalk that might inadvertently step out onto the street at a moments notice, and bike riders occasionally crossing in front of you as if they thought themselves invincible. With the stop signs, stop lights, and checking your rear view mirror, it is really amazing that we are able to do all those things at once without suffering accidents much more often. As a new driver you felt the stress while driving. After driving long enough it becomes second nature and you start to relax while driving.

A.D. is the same way, only in reverse. The things I used to do naturally, now demand a full conscious effort and intense concentration. This slows down everything I do. While I am in slow motion, time seems to pass faster than it ever did before. It is hard for me to keep up with the world's new pace, and it causes me great fatigue trying to stay in the present. I break projects down into small enough increments that I can actually complete something, one small step at a time. It is like taking baby steps, falling down and getting up again and again.

Most researchers and doctors believe that a person's IQ drops soon after being afflicted with A.D. I agree with this theory in part, but I don't know if my IQ has dropped because I no longer possess the ability to reason as well or only that it takes me longer to reason. Most of the IQ tests are timed, and I believe that if I were given an extended time period, I would perform as well as I ever did before. I believe that I can still, slowly, think complex, deeply, clearly, wisely, broadly...am I?

That would explain why A.D. victims are able to write much better than they can communicate verbally. However, I do agree that in the last stage of Alzheimer's, in which victims lose numerous abilities--conscious and unconscious ones--that their IQs are significantly lower and not just slower.

It is common for victims' math and spelling abilities to decline in stage one or two. I am currently losing ability in both of these areas. Sometimes, if I just wait a while, the answer will come, but other times, its just not there. My handwriting skills are also declining, but if I go very slowly I can still write legible. How does it feel to know I am losing my abilities? One aggravation is that I have had my Pre-A.D. abilities so long that they seem natural. So I have to unexpectedly confront my newly obtained limitations repeatedly each day. Maybe a good analogy would be that of an adult cat soon after being de-clawed. The cat will still often act as if he had claws. The cat doesn't realize his claws are absent and do not function properly until he attempts to use them and fails. Another example would be a person who had his legs amputated. For quite sometime after the operation, he may decide to get up from sitting in front of the television and start to do so, only to immediately be reminded of his condition. I am sometimes stunned upon re- discovering my diminished abilities, but I have been able to accept them so far.

Let me try to explain the concentration and energy that is required of me just to accomplish simple tasks. I'm sitting in my recliner, and I decide to get up from it. I have to consciously think to myself, the release lever is on the right, and then direct my arm to the release lever on the right, and hold onto it. Telling my leg to push down on the footrest at the same time I ask my arm to push down on the lever, while also preparing my back to lean forward. Some of my abilities fluctuate from moment- to -moment and day-to-day so it is hard to describe my typical degree of handicap. Usually I am about half way between the way I just described and what my normal was before A.D.

It is common for A.D. victims to fluctuate in their progression like I do. Some speculate that the cells ability to communicate properly improves at times. Some of the medicines prescribed for Alzheimer's disease victims are designed to improve cell communication. I have heard many testimonies to the benefits of these drugs from friends. There have been accounts of extreme fluctuations in which victims well into stage three of Alzheimer's disease, no longer able to recognize anyone and not aware of their surroundings, suddenly are able to recall their lives and to recognize others for a brief time. If the brain is basically destroyed in areas by these tangled fibers and webs, it does not seem likely that an improvement of that magnitude could occur. I suspect there is a way for the brain to re-route lost abilities. If that were proven to be true, perhaps one day we could learn how to improve the re-routing process. Another theory, although less probable, is that there is a psychic ability to recall things from parts of the mind that no longer function normally.

Another feeling I have, due to having Early Onset Alzheimer's disease, is an almost constant clouded mind. The best way I can describe this is perhaps how you might feel after taking a sleeping pill or after you have extremely exhausted yourself, but you can't rest yet. After a while I grew accustomed to this feeling and have been able to adapt and accept it without too much difficulty. I also have a feeling of complacency, like relaxing after a very long exhausting race. I don't wish to lay back and do nothing, but it's as if the competition is over for me. I can finally putt along at my own speed. I believe this feeling occurs in many other Alzheimer's disease victims, based on my discussions with them. Like me, some of A.D. victims have found that without the fear of failure they are free to take more risks and have gone on to try things, they would not have before having A.D.

I am often frustrated with myself because completing a task--composed of numerous minor tasks--requires so much effort and concentration. I force myself to focus on each stage as well as keeping track of the task as a whole. Take cooking a roast for instance. It would not matter how well I prepared the roast if I put it in the oven, and then took a nap to recoup the energy I expended in the process, if I forgot to turn the oven on.

Failing at one tiny piece of the task causes the entire task to be remembered as failure. This is extremely hard to deal with. My frustration is greatly increased when I am already disappointed in myself and someone else points out my ineptitude. The combination of failure and criticism discourages me from trying again. On the contrary, words of encouragement help me continue enduring. Often times it takes me two or more attempts to do even simple things like dialing a phone number. At times it makes me wonder if it is worth the effort anymore. I think many of us A.D. patients consider this, especially after making mistakes.

We can be so disappointed over letting a loved one down that it breaks our hearts. At times I wonder, is it worth it? Then I think what choice do I have? Eventually I stuff the hurt inside and force myself to go on for the sake of my loved ones. I realize that our loved ones are only human, and that our mood swings and inadequacies can extremely challenge their patience. Realizing that makes us feel even worse, for the strain we put on them. Barb has a T shirt that says: God has never failed me yet, but he sure comes very close. I think, we victims, and our loved ones, can all relate to that saying.

Several distortions of time and place occur to me. I can be driving someplace and all of a sudden I'm in a place much ahead of where I last remember being. I evidently lose memory of the miles I have just traveled. Sometimes the reverse happens and in my mind I think I am already past someplace but then I find myself just approaching it. It's like I am someone's doll and their large invisible hand reaches down, picks me up, and moves me to the place of its choice.

I often go blank, finding that I am somewhere I don't recognize or remember going to. I usually look around to figure out where I am, why I am there and where I am going. Why does this happen? Why does it only happen sometimes? I haven't been able to find or create a theory for that yet. This effect occurs as I am writing this book. It's like reading a story and accidentally turning two pages unknowingly. You can't figure out why you lost the continuity of the story. You continue to read and finally realize you must have skipped a page. This makes it very difficult to write this book. I can finish handwriting a sentence, and go blank. What did I just write? What topic was I on? I have to go back and read the last few pages to get back on track. The same thing happens on a larger scale; I forget what the previous chapter was about and have to refer back to the previous chapter to gather my thoughts and continue on properly. The more chapters I write, the harder it is to keep track of previous chapters. I use an outline of what I've done so far, but sometimes while reading the outline I forget the early sections before I complete reading the last section.

I can look right in the direction of something at times, but not see it. A while ago I was writing at the kitchen table. I thought I heard the phone but I could not see it. I asked my grandchildren if they knew where the phone was and my granddaughter, Natalia, walked over to the kitchen table and touched the phone. It was only inches away from me and even though I looked on the table for it, it was somehow invisible until she touched it. This happens to me quite often and I don't know why. How can I look at something and not see it, yet I see everything else right around it? It can be hard to deal with the strange powers of Alzheimer's disease, but I have no choice but to accept them and to keep on going.

I am writing this book as rapidly as possible. It is hard to do, and I am very slow at it, but I expect it to become continually harder all the time. I would go slower so I could do more research, but I'm afraid my ability to write would decline too far to complete it.

A Bit on My Death Sentence

Let me address what it was like to have my death sentence announced. Actually, everyone has been given a death sentence. The difference is that they haven't been given an approximate time in which they will face death. It was much easier for me to avoid thinking of my death when I had no idea of when it would occur or how. It was possible to mentally compartmentalize my life and view a very elderly person that would die in my place. Once I was diagnosed with Alzheimer's disease I was constantly reminded of my pending death sentence. It is attached to all of us with Alzheimer's disease and every time we can't think of a word, or we have difficulty doing things that used to be easy, we are reminded of our disease and all that accompanies it, including death. We spend every day aware that we are losing our minds and death is imminent. Many of us bear all this with as little fuss as possible, for the sake of our loved ones. Many of us try very hard not to burden our loved ones anymore that absolutely necessary. We understand some of what our loved ones are going through and want to spare them every burden possible. I sometimes think of how I would feel if my spouse had A.D instead of me. I truly believe I would be suffering more than I am now. I would probably try to deal with God by saying, "Please take this away from Barb, and let me have it in her place."

I am so sorry to have put my wife in this position. I take great consolation in the fact that soon she and I will be relieved of this burden and we will walk eternity together. If someone put a gun to us victim's heads and demanded we put this kind of hurt on our family, I'm sure many of us would refuse to do it. But A.D. doesn't give us a choice. It just commands that it be done...at least until we find a cure.

A Bit on Overcoming
my Death Sentence

When I was first diagnosed as having Early Onset Alzheimer's disease, I accepted it as factual and almost immediately started to prepare for my pending death. I just assumed that was how it worked. I had carried many Alzheimer's Disease victims to the ambulance or morgue, from nursing homes. I thought that once you get Alzheimer's disease, you spend a year or two out of your mind and then you die!

Since that time, I have studied Alzheimer's disease, and formed the opinion that I was wrong by a few years, but basically right. But then, I started reading books written by people with Alzheimer's disease. I could not comprehend how these people were able to do something like that years after their diagnosis of A.D. Eventually I communicated on the Internet with some D.A.S.N.I members, and finally spoke personally to some of these authors. Not all the members of D.A.S.N.I are writers, some where teachers, nurses and engineers and numerous other professions. After chatting with them and observing my own progression into Alzheimer's, it seems that each victim's attitude and will power actually slows or expedites the disease's progress. To really go out of a limb, I even wonder if it can be overcome indefinitely or at least until we die of unrelated causes. It may be wishful thinking, but at this point I am not sure that it isn't possible. I have met Alzheimer's disease victims who have been diagnosed 8-10 years ago and are still going strong (in a relative sense, of course). One thing I do know for a fact is will power and hope sure don't hurt, and any unconditional love given us serves as a power source for will power and hope.

CHAPTER 12
What We Want

Everyone has needs and desires. Alzheimer's disease limits its victim's ability to meet them, but it does not instantly eliminate all chances. Like everyone else, there will come a time when we can no longer help to satisfy our own desires and needs, but until that day we want to help ourselves and all of the Alzheimer's disease victims, as much as possible. We don't always get what we want, but neither does anyone else. What do most of us want? First and foremost we want to love and be loved. We desire good health, and economic security. We want to be useful and productive. We want to be accepted for who we are. We want the best for our families. We want to share in laughter and tears. We want to comfort, and to be comforted. We want fellowship with others who have Alzheimer's like us, and we want to see our children and grandchildren grow.

There are few, if any, people living that have all of these blessings in their fullness. We have all learned by now that what we want is not always what we get. We can try to change things for the better, but when that is not possible, we have two choices: to sulk over the immovable problem, or to attempt to adapt and overcome. This is a normal process in life that we all do or we become bitter and depressed. Those of us with Alzheimer's disease are often required to make adaptations. The adaptation we make can have an affect on others also. This is when we especially need the patience and cooperation of others. We understand how hard that can be on others, but we are not purposely doing it. It is being forced on us to.

Usually the "others" who have to accept our adjustments, are our close family members, in particular, our caregivers. They are given the opportunity to provide us with the greatest gift that can be given, as they accept our changes. That gift, "Unconditional Love" it is our absolute need. When we see it demonstrated by those who stand by us it is a source of our strength. It's our reason for pushing on. It's our weapon, which holds back the attacking enemy.

Even though we are slow, and not capable of everything we used to be able to do, we still want to be allowed to contribute in every way we can. Like everyone, we want to be allowed the opportunity to do everything we are still capable of. Depending on each individual's present condition, there are many things we are capable of doing. We often feel guilt for our inability to do more, and for the negative effects our disease has on our families emotionally, physically and financially, but that just makes us want to help even more. We only ask for your permission that we be allowed to help and be useful. Sharing and laughing together is a wonderful blessing. It's easy to get so wrapped up in our problems, that we forget the most precious things: sharing, loving, laughing, and hoping. Thank God for these things and enjoy them to their fullest. We don't want to be excluded from these things, so please count us in! Please don't consider us the breathing dead. We are still very much alive. Don't try to bury us, It Ain't Over Yet!

We want to be treated with respect by others. I don't think this is a common problem with those very close to us, but the general public tends to talk down to people with Alzheimer's Disease. Basically, I want them to know that we are slower, not dumber. I think the early to mid stages of Alzheimer's Disease should be called "Slow man's Disease." It does more to define the condition.

Fellowship with other Alzheimer's Disease victims is incredibly helpful. If you or your loved one with Alzheimer's are not involved in meeting with other victims of Alzheimer's Disease, I urge you to start as soon as possible. You can call your local chapter of the Alzheimer's Association, or contact D.A.S.N.I. Both of them can get you connected with the other. I am currently starting an Early Onset Alzheimer's Group in our area. Those of us with Early Onset Alzheimer's disease share some things in common with other Alzheimer's victims, but we have even more in common with Early Onset Alzheimer's Disease. Whether you have Alzheimer's or Early Onset Alzheimer's Disease, please get involved with a group of your peers as soon as possible. You will never regret it! Only a small percentage of Early Onset Alzheimer's, or A.D. victims ever become involved with other victims of the disease. This is a sad fact that need not be so. It is estimated that there are well over 2000 people with Early Onset Alzheimer disease within my home area of St. Louis, Mo. A.D. chapter. But to my knowledge less than a dozen or so participate or have any association with other Early Onset Alzheimer's Disease victims. There are many more thousands of A.D. victims in the same situation. I hope we can find a way to reach all those out there living with this disease, without any peer support.

The last desire I want to write about can be mistaken as negative or morbid, but it is not. Everyone alive today, old enough to know, realizes they will die one day. If you have a terminal disease like A.D. or cancer, you may feel closer to that day. This is not a subject to continually dwell on. Yet one should be prepared for its inevitable arrival. I pray that when that day comes for me, I have been allowed to live up to that day with faith, love, and dignity. I hope that the last expression my face ever makes is a smile. And I pray that if I go before my loved ones, God prepares them to willingly let me go. Rather than being a final deathblow, I want them to hear the sounding of the trumpet! CHARLEY IS GOING HOME! But we will meet again at God's appointed time.

CHAPTER 13
SPIRTUAL JOURNEY

I was a ten-year-old boy, taken to church on a regular basis since I was five years of age. It was then that I began having my first doubts about whether God existed. I had been taught about God in heaven and his son, Jesus, who died on the cross and rose again, so that we could have forgiveness for our sins but how could I know if it was true? If it wasn't true, I didn't want to dedicate my life to a myth. On the other hand, if God was truly alive, I didn't want to reject him. I decided to pray sincerely for a sign from God, verifying his existence. I told God that I was going to go downstairs to the bathroom, and when I flipped the switch to turn the light on, I wanted God to keep the light from turning on. I proceeded down the stairs and headed toward the bathroom at the end of the hall. I entered the bathroom and hesitated before reaching for the light switch. I readied myself to flip the light switch very nervously. My future rested on this one moment. I summoned up the will power, and slowly I flipped the light switch up. My stomach leapt to my throat; the room remained dark! What a miracle God had provided for this truly sincere young lad. I stood there in awe for a minute, and then a voice in my mind spoke to me. Maybe the light switch was broke, or the light bulb had burnt out. This was far too important of a decision to make if there was any doubt. Once again, I prayed sincerely to God, admitting my confusion. I prayed for the truth. I asked God to make the light turn on this time when I turned the light switch on again. I slowly flipped the switch off. It stayed dark. And then back on. I was amazed and filled with joy. God was real! He had made the light come on!

One would think that a miracle like that would convince a sincere seeker for a lifetime. But it was not over for this boy. I would be strongly influenced by experiences yet to come.

For the next two years I did my best to live for God. To me, living for God means letting my heart lead the way, treating others kindly, and doing my best to obey God's word. As the next few years passed I witnessed others in instance after instance blatantly disobeying God's word. It particularly bothered me that much of this behavior came from members and officials of the church. I knew that everyone had failures and that no one was perfect, but I saw behavior so blatant and repetitive--in total disregard for God--that I wondered if these people believed in God at all. Was church just a social club, were people just pretending to believe? Was it like a costume party where everyone dressed up and played their roles until the party was over? Had I been duped into building my whole life around a game they created for me to play? And to think, I had once thought of living my life for God, committing all of my time and energy toward serving Him, toward playing their game.

One day as a twelve-year-old boy gazing out the window, the dark side of life revealed itself to me. It was as if I had been blind and could now see things for what they truly were. It truly was an overwhelming experience. Suddenly, I saw the world, not as the loving place I once thought it to be, but full of self-serving people. I felt anger and sympathy simultaneously toward this new world. I was dazed and confused. How did I not see this before? Where had my deception come from? Was I alone in my new revelation? Grief filled me and all my crying did nothing to reduce the pain. I could now recall many things that pointed to evidence of a truly, sinister world. Had I somehow been protecting myself from recognizing the real world? I faced a dark new world, completely alone. A world where "love" was a word often used, but seldom truly meant. Depression consumed me for years after this revelation. The following year I spent alone as often as possible. I needed to know if this dark world was truly real or if I had somehow drawn the wrong conclusion. The more I observed the world from thereafter, the more it reinforced my idea of the world as a truly hurting place. My new view of the world caused me to question my religious beliefs once more. My entire belief system had crumbled. Was there truly a loving God? For the next eight years I would consider myself an agnostic. I continued to attend church to satisfy my parent's expectations, but I had lost my personal conviction. I even doubted the original miracle that God had given to me years earlier. I was old enough by then to know that a light switch could malfunction, work one time and not the next. Surely that must be what I had mistaken as a sign from God that he was real. After all, if God's own house didn't believe in him, how could he be real?

When I was fifteen I confronted my parents with my feelings. I told them that I could no longer pretend to believe. I refused to attend church with them any longer. My parents reluctantly conceded, and I did not attend church for many years.

I was sad, lonely, depressed and confused from the moment the doubting began. I wanted God to be real because I wanted to believe that good would conquer evil, and that love was stronger than greed and selfishness. Instead, my heart was filled with grief and anger for the way things were. I not only quit attending church but quit school as well. I joined the work force and continued to live with my grief. But God did not give up on me.

At sixteen years old I found, and soon married, the girl who would help me to restore my faith in love. We were ideal for one another. The girl had been deeply hurt by the divorce of her parents. Her faith in her dad had been shattered when she learned that he had been living a lie. He wasn't the husband or father she had thought him to be. Instead he was a womanizer who betrayed his own family. She needed someone she felt was strong enough to provide the sense of security she had recently lost. I needed someone who could show absolute loyalty and commitment. Although we had major differences, we fulfilled many of each other's needs. Sometimes our date time together was spent with Barb weeping on my shoulder as I held her and silently grieved over my own pain. We didn't know it then but we had entered into a time of healing.

We married, and continued healing our wounds. I saw true love displayed by my wife and slowly let her love tear down the barrier between God and myself. If love like God promised did exist, then there was hope that God existed also. Feeling loved by someone for the first time in my life, opened a path for me to receive God again.

When I was 20 I started reading the Bible again. A short time later God, once again impressed his reality on me. I committed myself to God in spite of all the phonies I knew of. I decided that just because some people, who call themselves children of God, did not believe, did not mean that God was not real. Never again could their behavior deter me from serving this wonderful God. My marriage bore fruit and we soon increased our small family. I was allowed to watch in the delivery room where I witnessed yet another miracle. The miracle of birth! A year and a half later, the miracle happened again!

We were so happy, serving a Living God, and having recently been blessed with two precious bundles of joy. How we loved our children, and all the troubled children and teens that we took into our home, usually temporarily. I was never very good at making money. I made poor business decisions, like quitting a high paying job because the boss was unfair to another employee. I started my own business and found that I was too softhearted to succeed as a business owner—but not until numerous attempts at it. By the time I was 28 I was deep indebt in part due to my generosity and sensitivity to other's situations. I decided to get a full-time job with reliable pay, and to run my business on the side. I wanted to use whatever talents God gave me to help others. I considered what my talents were. I was strong, knowledgeable of human behavior, calm in disasters and chaos, and sensitive to others feelings.

Convinced that I was adequately equipped to be a police officer, I started applying at local Police Departments. After filling out numerous, long, and tedious applications, and after several months, I had still not been hired anywhere. I thought that I might have made a mistake in choosing police work. I was ready to give up when a friend told me of a Department hiring. I haphazardly filled out the application only listing one or two of the various jobs I had held, and not adding details about them as I had done on the other applications. I figured that it didn't really matter. I hadn't been hired by anyone yet, so I was just going through the motions. Surprisingly I was hired and so began my new career. I was determined to maintain my commitment to God while working my new job, as I had in my previous jobs.

The exposure I received by doing police work in the 17th highest crime rate city per capita in the U.S. didn't take long to affect my behavior. I found that polite, clean language was interpreted as a sign of weakness in this area. I reasoned, that if using fowl language would prevent me from having to use force it was acceptable. My vocabulary changed but my heart remained committed to God. I was bothered by the minor illegal and unethical behavior some officers engaged in. But if the Chief was okay with it, what could I do about it? I found myself slowly hardening to ease the effects of the pain from observing the cruelty people continuously inflicted on one another. But I still felt that I was supposed to be there, so I gave it my all. Within a year I ranked with the top officers in arrests.

I had made some major arrests and gained the respect of even the most jaded officers along with an accommodation from the Chief. Still, something was happening inside me. I was becoming more and more callous.

I read my Bible and tried to apply what I had read to my job. I prayed over the dying, but they still died, over again and again until I started questioning the power of prayer and my interpretation of the Bible. The more money I made, the more my wife and I spent. Often it was spent to help others. So I worked about 50 hours a week at my part-time business, while still working full time at the police department. Throughout the remainder of my police career I worked at several different departments and grew increasingly calloused.

By now I seriously doubted my interpretation of the Bible because things didn't seem to happen the way the Bible said that they would. Convinced that ministers and church members were generally insincere, I questioned where I could find answers to my many spiritual questions. I got involved with a group that claimed to have the spiritual answers that I was seeking. But after joining their program and studying with them for several months, I recognized that they were leading me into a direction of evil and occult. I severed all connections with them, but I still didn't have any answers. Besides being spiritually confused, I was dealing with an increase of stress at my job and in my personal life.

In my early 30's my spiritual confusion and continued stress took its toll on me. I began having panic-attacks, with anxiety, heart palpitations, shortness of breath, and flue-like symptoms. The next year of my life seemed close to a living hell. I had to give up my business because I was too sick and weak to do the remodeling work. But I forced myself to continue with police work. I survived at my job by doing no more than was absolutely necessary, and as soon as my shift was over I would return home to bed. All year I prayed that God would heal me, or at least not let me slip deeper into my illness, mainly because I needed to continue caring for my family. I was sick, weak, and confused. I finally decided I had had enough. I told God that I was tired of asking for healing and stood ready to accept whatever God decided. I was too tired, sick and confused to continue on this way. I was broken in spirit. My mind had been affected. My memory had been severely damaged, and my body was weak. My cry out to God was my last effort to survive... or not. Once again, God miraculously intervened in my life! I began to heal, mentally, physically and spiritually. God had shown His patience and commitment to me, a confused but sincere young man. He blessed me with a peace I never thought possible during my healing. I never did solve all my spiritual questions, but I did find great peace brought on by His love. I learned to seek and to accept God's will. I prayed for God to keep me in His will, even if it meant death.

At fifty two years old I was diagnosed with Early Onset Alzheimer's disease. I am so thankful to God for giving me internal and eternal peace. God healed me and allowed me to raise my children. God even added a bonus of a son-in-law, daughter-in-law, and five precious grandchildren. I will not tempt the Lord God by pleading for another life extension. That's totally up to God. I am satisfied to let him decide.

CHAPTER 14
Caregivers

How does one thank another who has laid down their own desires to dedicate their life to being another's caregiver?

"Greater love hath no man than this that a man lay down his life for his friends"

I have tried to live my life adhering to this love letter, and I intend to continue doing so with all the strength I can, as long as I can. But the reality is that as I deteriorate I will be less capable of giving and become more and more dependent. This breaks my heart because I have found the true joy in giving, and to not be able to give is to cease existing for me. But I also realize that God wants to bless others with the joy of giving and he may intend on using me as a receiver so others may be blessed.

I am reminded of a true story about a young mentally-challenged man who was playing in a huge sand pile with a child. The sand pile started to collapse covering both of them. Rather than attempting to save himself, the young man focused his mentally challenged mind on saving the child. The sand reached the head of the young man and was slowly suffocating him. He continued to hold the child as high above his head as he could reach. He saved the child's life and sacrificed his own. Even as his very own breath was taken he continued to hold the child high, rather than struggle for his own life. In our culture today, we idolize professional athletes, movie stars, politicians, and financially successful people. I have refused to fall into that mode. To me the mentally challenged man in this story is out of their league. What a reward that must await this hero!

There was another young man, recently diagnosed as terminal. The Make a Wish Foundation, a non-profit organization that grants young terminal patients a wish like a trip to Disney World or to meet someone famous, granted this young man a "wish." He only asked for the opportunity to go with them and to participate in fulfilling the next person's wish. These are the kind of people who I respect. They are a rare find in our culture today, and I'm looking forward to meeting many of them in eternity.

Where do we find heroes like this? Those of us with Alzheimer's disease often have to look no further than to our caregivers, a loving, dedicated person who gives at the cost of a large portion of their own lives. I try to thank my caregiver and wife every opportunity I get. But there may come a day when I'm no longer thankful. There may be a time when I will insult and defy my caregiver. I know of many caregivers who are dealing with this, yet they continue to love and care for their Alzheimer's disease victim. What a grand example of self-sacrifice.

It brings me joy to think of the day when all their burdens will be lifted and they will receive a commendation from the Lord. They have truly earned it! Those of us with Alzheimer's disease never asked for this terrible disease, and once we found out that we had it we had only two choices: live with it or die. Our loved ones, turned caregivers, did not ask for us to have it either, but they have a choice. By choosing to stand by us, they are willingly surrendering themselves to the disease that we wish to run from. I don't know of any greater sacrifice, yet so many make the choice to join a loved one in this horrible illness.

Alzheimer's disease often creates a further openness for spiritual growth in its victims. I think this may be true with our caregivers also. While it greatly taxes them and they may often feel as though they can't go on, they do. And I think the process of pushing on furthers their spirituality. I can honestly say that I believe the caregiver's plight is worse than the victims.

In my career of firefighting, the media described my profession as heroic. I always felt uncomfortable with such claims. There were so many heroes in so many ways, and I never felt like firefighting deserved all the extra praise. Consider professions like, Police officers, carpenters, iron workers, evening and midnight shift convenient market cashiers, farmers, and so many others. These are all risky professions and many people are injured or killed working these jobs.

After the 9-11 tragedy occurred, much praise was given to the firefighting profession. But I want to tell you of an unsung hero. Shortly after the 9-11 tragedy, we responded to a 911 call of a child struck. Upon arrival we found an eleven year old boy lying in the street, where he had landed after being hit by a car. No matter how many tragic things emergency responders, firefighters, or police have seen it still breaks our hearts when a child's life is taken. The boy had been performing his duty as a school crossing guard when a car struck him. There were many victims that day, especially the parents of the child! What do you say to a parent at a time like that? After a day or two I got my thoughts together and decided to have a plaque made. It stated our Fire Depts. "Hero of the Year" award. We presented it to the parents and told them that their son had died in the line of duty, as he was protecting others' lives when his own was taken. I wished there was more I could do to help the parents, but I didn't know of any other way. I still pray for them whenever I recall the incident.

What about the single parent who works full-time, barely makes a living, raises their child or children, cleans house, cooks, entertains the child, and so on, every day over and over again? Yet they continue on and somehow maintain their sanity (mostly),while

having little or no time for interaction with other adults, except perhaps in a work environment. They are overworked, highly stressed, and often lonely, but they carry on with life. These are true heroes. I learned early in life that it is often necessary to stand completely alone, to follow my beliefs and live accordingly. I believe that sooner or later everyone will face a time when they have to be strong enough to stand alone, or compromise their conscience. Peer-pressure is a mighty force, and unless we develop the strength to stand alone when necessary, we will never be the person we truly want to be. There's a song I relate to, "I did it my way." I've heard this song criticized by some religious people. There reason being that a Christian should do it God's way, not his own way. I don't agree with that criticism. Because I interpret it to be saying that one must be strong enough to follow his convictions, with the strength God provides him. If your ways are God's ways, you will often need to be willing to stand-alone. Loneliness and enduring alone is a hard cross to bear, and often our caregivers subject themselves to this. Although as AD patients we are there physically, they observe more and more of our essence disappearing before their very eyes. Eventually, it reaches the point that they may feel alone even in our presence, as our ability to communicate deteriorates. The hurt and loneliness that I may inflict on my loved ones is the saddest part of my disease to me.

Mood swings are a symptom of Alzheimer's disease, so we victims may act Bi-Polar at times. There are times when I feel like I can beat this disease and avoid afflicting any further pain on others. Throughout my live there were many times that I had to summon up enough strength, determination, and will power, to confront and overcome tough situations. Today, as I write this section, I feel confident that I will defeat this disease's attempts to further hurt my loved ones. But I know that I am walking a tight rope and am barely balanced. I feel susceptible to falling off and becoming a further victim of the progression and depression of this destructive beast. I will resist this beast as long as I have the ability to do so. This is "my way," and as long as possible, I will continue to do it "my way."

I am exercising my right and commitment to do things my way in writing this book. I could seek advice and assistance from professionals to aid me in writing this book. But, if I did, they would probably ask me to change many things in it. Take the book cover for example. I use the word AINT, and the drawing is by my 12 yr old granddaughter, Jessicca. It's probably not what a large publisher or editor would accept. But it's my way; it's me. It's from my heart, and I feel it's the most honest way of expressing myself. So I will do it my way. I am so thankful that Barb understands this and supports me in it. She is a wonderful person and has already suffered many financial losses because of my strong convictions. Yet she never complained. No matter what the cost was, she understood. She has been my caregiver long before I had Alzheimer's disease.

I want to spare my loved ones the worst effects of this beast as long as possible. So I will resist it in every way I possibly can. By fighting back I am able to lesson some of the guilt I feel for subjecting them to the direct and indirect effects of my Alzheimer's. I want to whole-heartedly thank all the caregivers on behalf of myself--and those who no longer have the ability to do so. I truly don't have the words to properly express my gratitude. I don't think the words exist. But I want to at least say Thank You for being willing to stand alone, for having the courage to do it your way (GOD'S WAY)and for your love and dedication. And please forgive us, for at times we know not what we do.

CHAPTER 15
Fulfilling commitment

My outlook is considerably brighter today than the time immediately following my diagnosis. I am on retirement disability and have just been approved for social security disability benefits. I was a firefighter for the last seventeen years and a police officer for ten years prior to that. At times I loved my job, especially when I had the opportunity to help save people and their homes from fire, or to reunite a runaway child with his parents. But I was ready to leave that type work in the later years of my career. Both Police work and Firefighting expose you constantly to the saddest events in people's lives. I had observed far too much pain, hurt, suffering, hate and even death. I had reached the point that I wanted out. I would have liked a career change. Instead, my way out was through disability. God sure has a way of changing things.

Many people with Alzheimer's disease are disappointed that they have to abandon their careers. I honestly have to say,

I am glad to leave my career. I want to spend some time doing pleasant things.

When I began writing this book, I thought I had about one good year left, feeling there was no time to waste. Realizing how slowly I do things now, I have been fulfilling my commitments and making final preparations as rapidly as possible. My son is married now and off to a great start. God sent him a wonderful wife named Courtney. She has to be one of the kindest, compassionate ladies on Earth. As a result, I have gained a new daughter and two more precious grandchildren. Barb and I are living in a new home that I wanted to get for her, and she loves it. Most of the necessary legal and financial preparationsI needed to make are complete. I rented a pontoon boat and took the grandchildren fishing. Of course I let them operate the boat! My granddaughter, Jessicca, and I went to the Pine Ridge Indian Reservation and delivered the load of items for the needy that I had promised to supply. Of course we had to make the trip into a mini vacation. Jessicca and I share a love for Native Americans and many of their old ways. My brother, Rich, and his son Adam brought an additional truckload of supplies. We visited a fire breathing dinosaur, and Prairie Homestead with hundreds of white prairie dogs. My Granddaughter loved them and did not want to leave them. She loves all kinds of animals. Jessicca and Adam took a helicopter ride and climbed mountains in the Badlands. They really liked climbing the rocks and hills. I think their favorite part was dressing like cowboys in the 1880's town. Although I totally wore myself down and spent money I really couldn't afford, I am glad I did it. There just isn't any feeling better than watching children enjoy themselves. I have just about completed the projects I wanted to do for my mom, and I am now focused on preparing my family emotionally for my future decline and eventually departure to HEAVEN. Wont' that be a wonderful day when I can see Jesus face to face and all my loved ones that have gone their also? How great it will be.

I am writing this book partially to help prepare my family. I also hope this book will bring more understanding and comfort to those traveling the same road as me. Hopefully it will provide caregivers and everyone who knows someone affected by Alzheimer's, a better insight to what their loved ones are experiencing. Some times it is easier to write down how you feel than to tell it to the people that you should. There is a lot of literature to guide caregivers, but still very little literature written by people with Alzheimer's disease. One reason why few victims of Alzheimer's disease ever write a book is because they have often progressed too far in the disease by the time they are diagnosed, past the point of being able to perform a task that size. This is a sad fact and it need not be!

So often we ignore or deny the early symptoms while we loose valuable time. Time we could use to obtain new treatments. Time we could use to make future preparations. Somehow some way, the public needs to be informed of this common error. By confronting Alzheimer's disease sooner, victims could possibly prolong the effects of this terrible disease. It would lessen the load on caregivers and reduce the stress on loved ones. Between the day of my diagnosis of Alzheimer's and today, I have read much literature on Alzheimer's disease. And as I mentioned earlier, I was privileged to locate and read some books written by persons with this disease. I have been extremely uplifted by reading these books. I owe a deep debt of gratitude to those courageous individuals who pioneered this concept. All of the authors were victims of Early Onset Alzheimer's Disease. I suspect the reason why Early Onset Alzheimer's disease victims have written most, or all, of the books authored by Alzheimer's disease victims may be due to a couple of factors. The first reason may be that we are usually diagnosed nearer the start of the disease. Perhaps because we are usually still employed when Alzheimer's disease strikes us we have to confront its effects sooner, to attempt to deal with it. Most types of employment require the use of long and short-term memory. One of the earliest symptoms of Alzheimer's disease is short-term memory loss. As our short term memory loss increases it affects our job performance, eventually enough to force us to seek medical attention. On the contrary, an older, retired person can go without confronting the disease's effects longer with their sedentary lifestyle. Consequently, by the time they are diagnosed with Alzheimer's disease they are often well into Stage 2 of the disease, and their symptoms are too severe to deal with a task the size required to write a book. The second reason why I think us Early Onset Alzheimer's disease people have written more books is due to the difference in the situation of our lives when the disease strikes us. We are usually still employed and not financially prepared to retire. More is needed and expected of us due to our younger age. Feeling pressure to meet those needs may encourage us to push harder. Maybe the need to push on causes us to remain more active and resistant to the disease.

We often resist harder not because we are stronger, but because we feel forced too. If this is true, perhaps we should encourage all victims to resist more, slowing the effects of this terrible disease. But who, when, and how will we reach the many victims of this terrible disease?

I am presently a member of the group called D.A.S.N.I. that I referred to previously. It is an international organization, which supports people with all types of Alzheimer's disease and or Dementia. The group has an Internet chat room. I have met some wonderful, encouraging people with Alzheimer's disease and other forms of Dementia on this site. I had the privilege of meeting many other members of the group in person at a recent conference in Oklahoma. Some of them have had Alzheimer's for over 6 years and are still reasonably functioning. Some have actually improved in the last couple years. This was a great encouragement to me, and has changed my expectations of how long I may have left to reasonably function. We suspect that the medicine available now, coupled with our active resistance to Alzheimer's, may be the reason for our longevity.

When I started writing this book, I thought I had only a very short time to prepare for a rapid decline and ultimate death. I now expect that I may have five or ten more years, or possibly longer. With the possibility of reasonably functioning it's possible that God will extend my life once again. I am content to accept whatever time I have left, whether it is short or long. I have now realized there are many reasons why it may be beneficial to my loved ones and others for me to remain alive longer. I also want to help doctors, caregivers, and victims of Alzheimer's disease to understand that a diagnosis of Alzheimer's is not necessarily a rapid death sentence. I feel that many people diagnosed with Alzheimer's mentally surrender and allow the disease to rapidly overcome them. I want to do all I can with my remaining time to educate others of the potential they still have after being diagnosed with Alzheimer's disease.

I am truly excited about the extended time I may be given and have started planning future goals again. Instead of just planning for my rapid decline and death!

CHAPTER 16
THE PRESENT AND FUTURE

So here I am, perhaps, in the autumn of my life. As I wrote this book, I have mentally and emotionally relived much of my life. Through doing so, I have found that the sad times do not prevail over good memories. For example, the good memories of the joy I shared with our Jessica and the satisfaction of how my wife and I loved and tried to help her are very dominant over the hurt I felt when we lost her. I can relate it to something I frequently experienced with my children. One thing that comes to mind for example is when we took our children to a circus. They probably argued with each other, and wondered how long it would be until we got there. They complained if it didn't start after we got there, and no matter what we bought them, it never seemed to satisfy them. But a day or two later they would tell others how much fun they had there. It seemed the trivial displeasing memories were already forgotten.

I think this observation may be an insight into our own lives. When all is said and done, what remains are the memories of times we felt love and joy. Those negative things that sometimes overwhelmed us during our life's journey have greatly diminished in our minds. Life itself, and my survival, has been a demanding struggle, and although my body and mind have suffered the wear and tear that life dishes out, I can truly say the good times out weigh the bad. They remain dominant while others diminish. I know that with Alzheimer's disease there may come a time when I have few or almost no memories, but I suspect the good feelings will still be present. I cannot predict what temporary feelings, or lack there of, I may experience in the last stages of Alzheimer's disease, but I am confident that when it is finally over my God will wipe away the tears and we will rejoice together. I am so thankful for all the opportunities God has provided me to help others. Those times are some of my choice memories now, and I hope I continue to use every opportunity to continue doing so.

I am also very thankful for the family God has given me. I have been blessed with a loving wife who has, and will, stand by me always. Perhaps my greatest blessing of all is living long enough to see my wife, children, and grandchildren develop hearts of love and kindness. I cannot adequately describe the joy and satisfaction this brings me. Knowing that they are kind, caring, compassionate, loving children of God, gives me the greatest satisfaction that any human being could have.

These few written pages contain only a small portion of my life, thoughts, and feelings. There are so many other things I considered including. I feel somewhat guilty by not including or expanding on many thoughts and experiences. But, as I mentioned earlier, time is fleeting and I feel the need to complete this as expeditiously as possible. I am satisfied that what I have written will help provide you with some insight and understanding of the person with Alzheimer's Disease, and I'm grateful for being given the opportunity to contribute. AD patients die earlier than most, but until that time we need to be part of life's joys, decisions, love and all else that life offers. We may have Alzheimer's Disease, but, for many of us, It Still Aint Over Yet. We ask for your understanding and thank you for all you do. I have asked my wife to write the last chapter. She addresses the subject from a caregiver's perspective, and I feel it is proper that she has the last word.

May God bless you for caring and giving so much.

CHAPTER 17
Caretaker/Wife's
Story

The Doctor turned my world upside down when he came in to the office and said to my husband, "I don't have good news. You do not have MS, but you do have Alzheimer's Disease."

I didn't say anything for the next hour. I couldn't. Neither of us spoke a word on the ride home. Later, when I found my voice again, I kept repeating that it couldn't be true. We both decided it would be best not to tell our kids, or anyone, until we were certain. Charles didn't show any signs of Alzheimer's. He was still driving, thinking, and working. He was doing everything he had always done. But then, the more we thought about it, the more we realized how many signs we had ignored. Things started to make sense, like why he forgot and lost so many things and why he couldn't remember how he had gotten some place or how to get home.

Once we were certain that the diagnosis was correct, Charles asked me still not to tell anyone. He wanted to tell each person himself, when he was ready. It was constantly on my mind and I wanted to release some of the burden. Although I wanted to respect his wishes, I didn't like keeping this secret. I mentioned it to our daughter who was questioning me about her Dad's health. She agreed not to say anything to anyone. When Charles told her, a few months later, she let it slip that she already knew. My husband was very upset with me and refused to tell me certain things for months, reminding me that I couldn't be trusted.

Once I was free to relieve myself of the secret I had been shouldering, I was surprised how people reacted. Everyone took it better than I had expected, but that did not make things any easier. It actually made me feel more alone. I think, until this point, I still thought that someone was going to help me out of this predicament, and everyone's lack of concern meant that that was not the case. I would have to continue stomaching the bad news alone as it turned into a bad illness, supporting myself.

Charles and I are best friends, and I have always been able to depend on him. He was my rock. Now, I have to become more dependent on myself. I feel like a child who has gone somewhere new and, feeling frightened, hangs on to what they do know tighter. What I would hang onto is Charles. He comforted me when I felt intimidated by the colossal world.

I am losing my friend, who I could laugh with, cry with, yell at, who always watched out for me. Then I think of all that he is losing, like seeing our grandkids marry, their school graduations, college graduation, and great-grandchildren. I was angry with God for letting this happen, and I felt sorry for myself, crying privately. I felt guilty for all the times that I had yelled or said hurtful things, not realizing that he actually couldn't help it.

I had always been an early riser who moved all day long and crashed at the end of the day, waking up refreshed. But I began sleeping in whenever I could and was exhausted when I had to get up to work or to take care of chores. I just felt like I had no control over the outcome of my day and didn't know where to begin to fix it.

Six months after the diagnoses we signed up for an Alzheimer's Association membership. They screened us and decided we would fit well in their program, including a support group of 12 Alzheimer's patients and their spouses or caregivers. I sometimes felt that even though the people that I met were nice, that they couldn't understand my situation because it was so different from theirs. Unlike the rest of the members, my husband and I still worked. He also had other illnesses that prevented some of their advice -- taking walks together — from helping us. But I did get a chance to see that though these people were further along in their Alzheimer's, they were still individuals and not the horrid images a year of working in a nursing home had given me.

Eventually I got over the dismay of losing my husband to this disease. God blessed me with the strength I needed. I thought about how fortunate I was to have had time with Charles. I recognized that not too many people are given time to prepare for their departure from this world. Together, my husband and I have watched the grandkids grow, have seen our children marry, have spent time with family, and have vacationed together, even visited foreign countries spreading the gospel. God has really blessed us, and I'm so glad for all the times we had and for what we have right now.

Charles doesn't remember a lot of the past, good or bad. We have home movies and pictures I use to help remind him. He relives it as he watches it on the video. Often I have to tell him the same thing every five minutes. I try to remember that he can't remember, but there are those times when I get upset and frustrated by having to answer the same question over and over. I may lash out, and tell him that I have already answered that question. But he is not doing it to aggravate me; he just doesn't remember.

It is hard to start making all of the decisions myself after so many years of his help in making decisions. It is one of the hardest things about this disease for me. I have always second-guessed my own decisions, and Charles would step in and make the final one, while I waited to follow his lead. He is not as firm in his decisions as he used to be. He even calls me sometimes at work to ask my opinion. Other times he gets an idea in his head and insists on making a permanent decision right then. When that happens, I ask him to think about, and to talk to me about it later. Sometimes he changes his mind or forgets about it on his own. It scares me when I think of making important decisions all alone, but I know that I am not alone. God is there, and he helps me and guides me, just like he has guided Charles. So in a way it has made my trust in God stronger. I used to depend on my husband to listen to God for the both of us. Now, I pray more and question if I am following God's will.

Sometimes I feel bad if I want to go out and visit with friends or our daughter and daughter-in-law. Charles is always so wonderful. He encourages me to go and to have fun. He doesn't keep me attached to him all the time. He still lets me enjoy my life. I'm a very talkative, out-going person. Charles, on the other hand, is very quiet and doesn't like groups or lots of people. I've noticed that he likes crowds even less now that he has Alzheimer's disease, but he tries for me. When the stimulation becomes too much for him, he finds a deserted place somewhere. I have to remind myself that he can only do one thing at a time. I usually do the driving now, so that Charles can talk with me when we are in the car.

It seems like nearly everything he does takes three times longer than it would take me to do it for him. I try to be patient and to let him do it himself because I don't want to take away the little independence that he has left. Sometimes I have to fix the things that he does, sometimes he gets it, but sometimes I am not sure if it is right or not. I have to leave him notes or call him to make sure he is okay, or check that he has done what he needed to get done for that day. He has a cell phone, and that is how I usually get in contact with him. Most of the time he has his brother with him. He doesn't usually do things by himself, which is good. I don't worry as much when Charles is with someone.

For the most part, I have not been too worried about leaving him home alone. But one day I called home from work and there was no answer. I called his cell phone and got no answer there, so I left a message. I thought that his cell phone might be out of range, and that there was nothing to worry about. When I got off of work I called again, still no answer. Now I was becoming worried. I headed straight home, calling again and again, still no answer at the house or on the cell phone. I then tried a friends shop. They were not at his place either. Now I was really worried. It was about two hours after I got home when I finally heard from him. His brother and him were at an auction and didn't hear the phone. I told him that we had to make some changes. So he agreed, and we did. I turned up the volume on his cell phone and made it vibrate. I told him I was going to enroll him in "safe return".

Charles is still alert and realizes how much he can't do, and how that affects me. I try to be tolerant and to remember that even though he does not appear to be sick at times, he is. There is a part of me that thinks it is just not fair that due to his other health problems he can't cut the grass or help me clean. A part of me has questioned why it is that he can't remember to put away his dirty dishes or to pick up his stuff, but he can figure out how to chat on the Internet. I feel like a single parent, working and running the house all by myself. I just have to accept what things are and let go of the unfairness of it all.

We do and have done so much with each other, but now it means so much more than it ever did before. I try to make sure he does as much as he can with the grandkids. He sees them a lot and goes places with them. He really enjoys spending time with them. We call these times our "memory making" times. They will always have their memories of Grandpa and how much he loved them and doing things with them. No one will be able to steal that away from them, even if the Alzheimer's takes away the Grandpa who they laughed and talked with. I know that someday his body may still be here but not his mind. So I try to enjoy each moment and hold on to it. It is a priceless gift, having time to prepare for our loss. Most people are not so lucky.

Charles is still here in body and in mind most of the time. He wants to keep busy, and he tries so hard to achieve many things. Bless his big wonderful heart. All of his life he has only thought of others. He is still doing that today. He worries about my finances and has planned well for me after his death. It will be very hard without him, but I wouldn't trade one day of what we had for anything.

Everyone copes differently, but my prayer is that you do everything you can to make what time you and your loved one have left a time to remember, something that when you look back you can say "I did all I could to make the time they had left a grand one."

I try to keep in mind that our days together are numbered. I am glad for each one that I have with him. I am not worried about his death. I feel it is selfish to do so just because we will all miss him so much. I plan to make each day we are given as wonderful as possible.

I don't know how I will handle it when his body is here but his mind has gone on. I pray that I don't have to find out, but I know that when, and if, it comes to that, my Lord will carry me through. I pray you will allow him to carry you too.

ABOUT THE AUTHOR

At fifty-two years old his career in public safety ended rather abruptly. A tenacious individual always ready to stand against injustice and aggression, a man who lived by wit, grit, and determination that allowed him to back his commitment to justice, even when he seemingly stood alone in them - now he is forced into battle for his very life, or worse, his mind. His previous battles now seem dwarfed by the magnitude of his present attacker. Realizing that his assets of wit, grit and determination may diminish as Alzheimer's Disease attacks his mind, he appeals for strength from his soul and through his faith. He is determined to continue to be as productive as possible. A native of St. Louis, Mo., happily married with two adult children and five grandchildren, his present desire is to continue to make memories with his family, encourage others, and promote a greater understanding of Alzheimer's Disease by writing and publically speaking as long as he is capable. He may be contacted at charley3rd@yahoo.com.

LaVergne, TN USA
18 March 2010
176401LV00003B/69/A